Copyright ©

1

Table of Contents

INTRODUCTION 4

Mediterranean diet 6

Is the Mediterranean Diet Still Good for You 7

What Are the Health Benefits of the Mediterranean Diet 9

What Foods Are Included in the Mediterranean Diet........... 10

The Importance of Olive Oil... 11

Benefits of the Mediterranean Diet 14

Healthy Mediterranean Diet Recipes 24

Zucchini Noodles with Marinara Sauce Recipe 25

Cancer-fighting foods 26

Cancer-Fighting Foods vs. Cancer-Causing Foods 30

Cancer-Fighting Foods 35

Other Ways to Increase Effectiveness of An Anti-Cancer Diet
.... 45

Cancer-Fighting Foods Recipes.. 54

Mediterranean diet for cancer 56

Evidence research... 56

Cancer prevention 56

Breast cancer 57

Colorectal cancer... 59

Other cancer types 60

Mechanisms of Action 60

Mediterranean Anti-Cancer Recipes 65

Red cabbage and walnut slaw 67

Cherry tomato pie 72

Lentil moussaka 77

Mushroom orzotto 78

Homemade tomato ketchup 82

INTRODUCTION

When our patients come to us with the goal of preventing cancer or cancer recurrence, our job is to help them optimize their nutrition, lifestyle, and environment. Food is consumed several times throughout the day, making diet one of the most important factors in the goal of influencing the body's biochemistry and physiology. While specific "super-foods" exist with well-studied phytochemicals, establishing healthy eating patterns is more important to influence overall health. The Mediterranean diet is a simple eating pattern that has gained popularity in recent years, being recommended in the 2015-2020 Dietary Guidelines for Americans. Adherence to a Mediterranean diet is associated with a decrease in chronic diseases such as cardiovascular disease, neurodegenerative disorders such as Alzheimer's and Parkinson's diseases, diabetes mellitus, and cancer. This book reviews the research that shows a correlation between the Mediterranean diet and a decrease in cancer incidence, the mechanisms that may explain the decrease, specific dietary goals to discuss with your patients, how to evaluate adherence to the Mediterranean diet, methods for improving bioavailability of nutrients, and adherence to this dietary pattern.A healthy diet plays an important role in primary and secondary prevention of cancer. The Mediterranean diet is associated with lower risk of several chronic diseases, including cardiovascular disease, neurodegenerative disease, diabetes, and cancerespecially cancers of the breast and colon. The mechanisms responsible for these effects include reductions in inflammation, oxidative damage, metabolic syndrome, and weight. The Mediterranean diet consists primarily of fish, vegetables, legumes, whole grains, potatoes, fruits, extra virgin olive oil (EVOO), moderate amounts of wine, and small amounts of red meat. It limits processed foods and refined sugar. Achieving this dietary pattern is a simple and attainable goal. Certain food preparation techniques can improve the bioavailability of important nutrients in the Mediterranean diet. Observational and clinical studies show the Mediterranean diet is effective for primary and possibly secondary prevention of cancer.

The "Mediterranean diet" represents the food consumed in about 16 countries bordering the Mediterranean Sea. Accumulating evidence points to the many health benefits conferred by this diet.

The diet consists of olive oil rich in monounsaturated fats, nuts, and fish, all excellent sources of omega-3 fatty acids, plus antioxidant-rich fruits and vegetables. It has been shown to reduce the risk of heart disease, cancer, and the incidence of neurodegenerative disorders such as Alzheimer's and Parkinson's disease. According to the American Heart Association, in addition to consuming a healthy diet and engaging in physical activity, social networks are also essential for disease prevention.

Mediterranean diet

Not only is the Mediterranean diet a tasty way to eat, drink and live, but it's also a realistic and sustainable way to reduce disease-causing inflammation and to lose weight, too (or to maintain a healthy weight). In fact, in January 2019 when U.S. News evaluated 41 of the most popular diets they identified the Mediterranean Diet as being the "#1 Best Overall Diet."

The Mediterranean diet has long been one of the healthiest diets known to man. The history and tradition of the Mediterranean diet come from the historic eating and social patterns of the regions around southern Italy, Greece, Turkey and Spain. Therefore the Mediterranean diet is really not even a "diet" in the way we usually think of them, more like a life-long way of eating and living. For thousands of years people living along the Mediterranean coast have indulged in a high-fiber diet of fruits and vegetables, also including quality fats and proteins in moderation, and sometimes a glass of locally made wine to complete a meal, too.

Meanwhile, this eatin pattern has gotten a reputation for disease prevention, mood-enhancement, and even "enjoyable" weight manageable. That's right, studies show the same diet that can help you shed excess weight, and keep it off too, can also reduce your risk for depression, cardiovascular disease and more.

Starting in Italy thousands of years ago and spreading to Greece, Spain and other areas around the Mediterranean, this diet is now successful all over the world for promoting health and longevity. While it's always existed, even before books and studies were dedicated to it, the diet really began to take hold around the world in the 1990s, when a Harvard University doctor showcased it as a diet useful for improving heart health, losing weight and clearing up other health issues.

Is the Mediterranean Diet Still Good for You

In 2013, a landmark study of more than 7,000 people in Spain was published. The study's subjects were split into three groups: those receiving advice about following a Mediterranean diet and getting extra-virgin olive oil delivered to their home; receiving advice about following the Mediterranean diet and getting nuts delivered to their home; and, in the control group, receiving advice about following a low-fat diet.

The study found that those people eating a Mediterranean diet that was supplemented with the olive oil deliveries were 30 percent less likely to die of heart attack, disease, stroke or death from cardiovascular causes than those eating a low-fat diet.In fact, the study finished earlier than planned, because the results were drastic enough that it was considered unethical to continue conducting it. For those of us who advocate eating a Mediterranean diet, this study was a welcome validation.

But in June 2018, the authors took the rare step of retracting the original study in the New England Journal of Medicine based on flaws in how the original study was conducted. It turns out that about 15 percent of the people in the study weren't actually placed in a particular group randomly people with a family member also participating were placed in the same group; one clinic assigned everyone to the same group; and another study site didn't properly use the randomization table.

The study's authors have said that after excluding the non-randomized people from the study and reexamining the data, the results still hold true. But because the study wasn't truly random, it can no longer claim that the health benefits are directly caused by the Mediterranean diet and olive oil.

Instead, a revised version of the study was released on June 13, 2018. This updated study made statistical adjustments to the data, accounting for the fact that it wasn't 100 percent random. The language is softer, too instead of saying that the Mediterranean diet was the direct cause of the reduced rate of cardiovascular diseases and death, it simply says that people following the diet had fewer instances of it.

So is the Mediterranean diet still healthy? Absolutely. While this one study may have been flawed, it doesn't change the fact that fresh fruits, veggies, lean proteins, whole grains, fish and healthy fats like olive oil (along with the occasional glass of wine!) are all foods that are proven to be good for you on their own. Together, they comprise a diet that can be terrific for your health study or no study.

What Are the Health Benefits of the Mediterranean Diet

Considered by many nutrition experts to be one of the most heart-healthy ways of eating there is, the base of the Mediterranean diet is loaded with anti-inflammatory foods and built upon plant-based foods and healthy fats.

Based on much research, this particular diet can protect against the development of heart disease, metabolic complications, depression, cancer, type-2 diabetes, obesity, dementia, Alzheimer's and Parkinson's. The best part is, even with all of these benefits, it still provides the opportunity for people to "eat, drink and be merry."

Ever wonder why people from the Mediterranean region seem so happy and full of life? It's tempting to attribute their good health and positive moods to one single factor alone like their diet, for example but the truth is that it's a combination of their lifestyle factors and their unprocessed diets that has promoted their longevity and low rates of disease for centuries.

According to the Harvard School of Public Health,"Together with regular physical activity and not smoking, our analyses suggests that over 80 percent of coronary heart disease, 70 percent of stroke, and 90 percent of type 2 diabetes can be avoided by healthy food choices that are consistent with the traditional Mediterranean diet."

What Foods Are Included in the Mediterranean Diet

The Mediterranean way of eating promotes foods including:

fresh fruits and vegetables (especially leafy greens like spinach and kale and non-starchy veggies like eggplant, cauliflower, artichokes, tomatoes and fennel) olive oil

nuts and seeds (like almonds and sesame seeds used to make tahini)

legumes and beans (especially lentils and chickpeas used to make hummus)

herbs and spices (like oregano, rosemary and parsley)

whole grains

eating wild-caught fish and seafood at least twice a week

high quality pasture-raised poultry, eggs, cheese, goat milk, and probiotic-rich kefir or yogurt consumed in moderation

red meat consumed on special occasions or about once weekly

plenty of fresh water and some coffee or tea

oftentimes a daily glass of red wine

The Importance of Olive Oil

Nearly every nutritional researcher attributes at least some of the legendary health benefits of the Mediterranean diet to the copious amounts of olive oil included in almost every meal. Olives themselves are an ancient food, and olive trees have been growing around the Mediterranean region since about 3,000 B.C.

Olive oil joins foods containing omega-3 fats, like salmon and walnuts, for example, as an elite category of healthy fatty acids. Olive oil has a ton of research backing its health benefits — in fact, it's so backed by research that the FDA even permits labels on olive oil bottles containing a specific health claim (to date this is only allowed on olive oil, omega-3 fats and walnuts). That claim?

Limited and not conclusive scientific evidence suggests that eating about 2 tablespoons (23 grams) of olive oil daily may reduce the risk of coronary heart disease due to the monounsaturated fat in olive oil. To achieve this possible benefit, olive oil is to replace a similar amount of saturated fat and not increase the total number of calories you eat in a day.

So what is it about olive oil that makes it so good for you?

To start, olive oil is very high in compounds called phenols, which are potent antioxidants capable of lowering inflammation and fighting free radical damage. Olive oil is mainly made up of monounsaturated fatty acids, the most important of which is called oleic acid. Oleic acid is known to be extremely heart-healthy in numerous ways, especially when compared to many other refined vegetable oils, trans-fats or hydrogenated fats.

Olive oil even has a step up in terms of heart health benefits compared to most grain-based carbohydrates — for example, high monounsaturated fat diets lower LDL cholesterol, raise HDL cholesterol and lower triglycerides better than carb-heavy diets do, according to some some studies.

How much olive oil should you consume daily? While recommendations differ depending on your specific calorie needs and diet, anywhere from one to four tablespoons seems to be beneficial. Estimates show that those in the Mediterranean region probably consume between three to four tablespoons a day, and this is the amount that some health practitioners recommend to their heart disease patients.

Just remember that all olive oil is not created equally. Unfortunately, most commercial manufacturers that are trying to ride the health hype on olive oil have rushed to the market with all kinds of fake olive oils, which are imitations and inferior products. The problem is these oils aren't always harvested or processed properly, which can kill many of their delicate nutrients and turn some of their fatty acids rancid or toxic.

Here's what really makes a big difference: Look for labels that indicate your oil is "extra-virgin" and ideally cold-pressed. Olive oil is almost unique among oils in that you can consume it in its crude form without any processing needed (for example, you could literally press olives and enjoy their natural oils).

While it's delicate and not necessarily the best oil for cooking, cold-pressed or expeller-pressed oil hasn't been refined so it holds all of its natural vitamins, essential fatty acids, antioxidants and other nutrients better. While unrefined oil is separated without high heat, hot water, solvents and left unfiltered, on the flip side some oils are heated to a high degree, which reduces their benefits.

Benefits of the Mediterranean Diet

1. Low in Processed Foods and Sugar

The diet primarily consists of foods and ingredients that are very close to nature, including olive oil, legumes like peas and beans, fruits, vegetables, unrefined cereal products, and small portions of animal products (that are always "organic" and locally produced). In contrast to the typical American diet, it's very low in sugar and practically free of all GMOs or artificial ingredients like high fructose corn syrup, preservatives and flavor enhancers. For something sweet, people in the Mediterranean enjoy fruit or small quantities of homemade desserts made with natural sweeteners like honey.

Beyond plant foods, another major staple of the diet is locally caught fish and a moderate consumption of cow, goat or sheep cheeses and yogurts that are included as a way to receive healthy fats and cholesterol. Fish like sardines and anchovies are a central part of the diet, which usually is traditionally lower in meat products than many Western diets today.

While most people in the Mediterranean aren't vegetarians, the diet promotes only a small consumption on meats and heavier meals — instead going for the lighter and healthier fish options across the board. This can be beneficial for those looking to lose weight and improve things such as their cholesterol, heart health and omega-3 fatty acid intake.

2. Helps You Lose Weight in a Healthy Way

If you're looking to lose weight without being hungry and maintain that weight in a realistic way that can last a lifetime, this might be the plan for you. The diet is both sustainable and worthwhile, and has been undertaken by many people all around the world with great success related to weight loss and more, as it works to help manage weight and reduce fat intake naturally and easily due to eating many nutrient-dense foods.

There's room for interpretation in the Mediterranean diet, whether you prefer to eat lower carb, lower protein or somewhere in between. The diet focuses on consumption of healthy fats while keeping carbohydrates relatively low and improving a person's intake of high-quality protein foods. If you refer protein over legumes and grains, you have the option to lose weight in a healthy, no-deprivation-kind-of-way with a high amount of seafood and quality dairy products (that simultaneously provide other benefits like omega-3s and often probiotics).

Fish, dairy products and grass-fed/free-range meats contain healthy fatty acids that the body needs, working to help you feel full, manage weight gain, control blood sugar, and improve your mood and energy levels. But if you're more of a plant-based eater, legumes and whole grains (especially if they're soaked and sprouted) also make good, filling choices.

3. Improves Heart Health

Research shows that greater adherence to the traditional Mediterranean diet, including plenty of monounsaturated fats and omega-3 foods, is associated with a significant reduction in all-cause mortality, especially heart disease. A striking protective effect of a Mediterranean diet rich in alpha-linolenic acid (ALA) from olive oil has been shown in many studies, with some finding that a Mediterranean-style diet can decrease the risk of cardiac death by 30 percent and sudden cardiac death by 45 percent.

Research from the Warwick Medical School also shows that when high blood pressure is compared between people eating more sunflower oil and those consuming more extra-virgin olive oil, the olive oil decreases blood pressure by significantly higher amounts.

Olive oil is also beneficial for lowering hypertension because it makes nitric oxide more bioavailable, which makes it better able to keep arteries dilated and clear. Another protective element is that it helps combat the disease-promoting effects of oxidation and improves endothelial function. Keep in mind that low cholesterol levels are worse than high sometimes, but people in the Mediterranean don't usually struggle to maintain healthy cholesterol levels either since they obtain plenty of healthy fats.

4. Helps Fight Cancer

According to the European Journal of Cancer Prevention,

The biological mechanisms for cancer prevention associated with the Mediterranean diet have been related to the favorable effect of a balanced ratio of omega-6 and omega-3 essential fatty acids and high amounts of fiber, antioxidants and polyphenols found in fruit, vegetables, olive oil and wine.

A plant based diet, one that includes lots of fruits and vegetables, is the cornerstone of the Mediterranean diet, which can help fight cancer in nearly every way — providing antioxidants, protecting DNA from damage, stopping cell mutation, lowering inflammation and delaying tumor growth. Many studies point to the fact that olive oil might also be a natural cancer treatment and decrease the risk of colon and bowel cancers. It might have a protective effect on the development of cancer cells due to lowered inflammation and reduced oxidative stress, plus its tendency to promote balanced blood sugar and a healthier weight.

5. Prevents or Treats Diabetes

Evidence suggests that the Mediterranean diet serves as an anti-inflammatory dietary pattern, which could help fight diseases related to chronic inflammation, including metabolic syndrome and type 2 diabetes. (9) One reason the Mediterranean diet might be so beneficial for preventing diabetes is because it controls excess insulin, a hormone that controls blood sugar levels, makes us gain weight and keeps the weight packed on despite us dieting.

By regulating blood sugar levels with a balance of whole foods — containing healthy fatty acids, quality sources of protein and some carbohydrates that are low in sugar — the body burns fat more efficiently and has more energy too. A low-sugar diet with plenty of fresh produce and fats is part of a natural diabetic diet plan.

According to the American Heart Association, the Mediterranean diet is higher in fat than the standard American diet, yet lower in saturated fat. It's usually roughly a ratio of 40 percent complex carbohydrates, 30 percent to 40 percent healthy fats and 20 percent to 30 percent quality protein foods. Because this balance is somewhat ideal in terms of keeping weight gain and hunger under control, it's a good way for the body to remain in hormonal homeostasis, so someone's insulin levels are normalized. As a byproduct, it also means someone's mood is more likely to stay positive and relaxed, energy levels up, and physical activity easier.

The Mediterranean diet is low in sugar, since the only sugar present usually comes from fruit, wine and the occasional locally made dessert. When it comes to drinks, many people drink plenty of fresh water, some coffee and red wine, too. But soda and sweetened drinks aren't nearly as popular as they are in the U.S.

While some Mediterranean diets do include a good deal of carbohydrates — in the form of pasta or bread, for example — being active and otherwise consuming very low levels of sugar means that insulin resistance remains rare in these countries. The Mediterranean style of eating helps prevent peaks and valleys in blood sugar levels, which zaps energy and takes a toll on your mood. All of these various factors contribute to this diet's diabetes prevention capabilities.

Most people in the Mediterranean eat a balanced breakfast within one to two hours of waking up, which starts their day right by balancing blood sugar when it's at its lowest. They then typically eat three meals a day that are filling, with plenty of fiber and healthy fats. Many people choose to have their biggest meal mid-day as opposed to at night, which gives them the opportunity to use that food for energy while they're still active.

You can see how this differs from the standard American diet, which often results in many people skipping breakfast, snacking throughout the day on energy-zapping foods high in carbs and sugar, and eating a lot at nighttime while they're sedentary.

6. Protects Cognitive Health and Can Improve Your Mood

Eating the Mediterranean way might be a natural Parkinson's disease treatment, a great way to preserve your memory, and a step in the right direction for naturally treating Alzheimer's disease and dementia. Cognitive disorders can occur when the brain isn't getting a sufficient amount of dopamine, an important chemical necessary for proper body movements, mood regulation and thought processing.

Healthy fats like olive oil and nuts, plus plenty of anti-inflammatory veggies and fruits, are known to fight age-related cognitive decline. These help counter the harmful effects of exposure to toxicity, free radicals, inflammation-causing poor diets or food allergies, which can all contribute to impaired brain function. This is one reason why adherence to the Mediterranean diet is linked with lower rates of Alzheimer's.

Probiotic foods like yogurt and kefir also help build a healthy gut, which we now know is tied to cognitive function, memory and mood disorders.

7. Might Help You Live Longer!

A diet high in fresh plant foods and healthy fats seems to be the winning combination for longevity. Monounsaturated fat, the type found in olive oil and some nuts, is the main fat source in the Mediterranean diet. Over and over, studies show that monounsaturated fat is associated with lower levels of heart disease, cancer, depression, cognitive decline and Alzheimer's disease, inflammatory diseases and more. These are currently the leading causes of death in developed nations — especially heart disease.

In the famous Lyon Diet Heart Study, people who had heart attacks between 1988 and 1992 were either counseled to follow the standard post-heart attack diet advice, which reduces saturated fat greatly, or told to follow a Mediterranean style. After about four years, follow-up results showed that people on the Mediterranean diet experienced 70 percent less heart disease — which is about three times the reduction in risk achieved by most cholesterol-lowering prescription station drugs! The people on the Mediterranean diet also amazingly experienced a 45 percent lower risk of all-cause death than the group on the standard low-fat diet.

These results were true even though there wasn't much of a change in cholesterol levels, which tells you that heart disease is about more than just cholesterol. The results of the Lyon Study were so impressive and groundbreaking that the study had to be stopped early for ethical reasons, so all participants could follow the higher-fat Mediterranean-style diet and reap its longevity-promoting payoffs.

8. Helps You De-stress and Relax

Another influencing factor is that this diet encourages people to spend time in nature, get good sleep and come together to bond over a home-cooked healthy meal, which are great ways to relieve stress and, therefore, help prevent inflammation. Generally, people in these regions make sure to spend a lot of time outdoors in nature; eating food surrounded by family and friends (rather than alone or on-the-go); and put aside time to laugh, dance, garden and practice hobbies.

We all know that chronic stress can kill your quality your life along with your weight and health. Those who practice the diet have the luxury of leisurely dining at a slow pace, eating local delicious foods almost every day and engaging in regular physical activity too — other important factors that help maintain a happy mood.

In addition, the history of the Mediterranean diet includes a love for and fascination with wine — especially red wine, which is considered beneficial and protective in moderation. For instance, red wine may help fight obesity, among other benefits. This smart choice of a healthy way of life leads to longer lives free of chronic complications and diseases related to stress, such as those caused by hormonal imbalances, fatigue, inflammation and weight gain.

9. Can Help Fight Depression

A 2018 study published in the journal Molecular Psychiatry found evidence that healthy dietary choices, those in line with eating the Mediterranean diet, can help reduce the risk for depression.Researchers involved in the study investigated the mental-health effects of adherence to a range of diets including the Mediterranean diet, the Healthy Eating Index (HEI), the Dietary Approaches to Stop Hypertension diet (DASH diet), and the Dietary Inflammatory Index. They found that the risk of depression was reduced the most when people followed a traditional Mediterranean diet and overall ate a variety of anti-inflammatory foods.

What is it about anti-inflammatory foods that helps boost your mood and mental health? Inflammation is frequently named as the root cause of many mood and psychiatric conditions, including schizophrenia, obsessive compulsive disorder, depression, anxiety, fatigue, and social withdrawal. The same lifestyle habits that tend to activate inflammation such as a poor diet, chronic stress and sleep deprivation also tend to produce brain states that contribute to mental illness. A nutrient-dense diet seems to help directly protect parts of the brain, while other dietary/lifestyle changes like getting good sleep, having a mindful approach to meals, planning meals ahead of time, and limiting stress can also lead to a calmer mindset.

Healthy Mediterranean Diet Recipes

Ready to get started eating in the same way as those living in the region? Here are some simple Mediterranean diet recipes for including more vegetables, fish, legumes, fruit, herbs and quality proteins in your diet:

Zucchini Noodles with Marinara Sauce Recipe

This Zucchini Noodles with Marinara Sauce Recipe is a great raw recipe full of flavor, fiber and vitamin C! Try this raw recipe for dinner tonight.

Total Time: 20 minutes

Serves: 4–6

INGREDIENTS:

- 2–4 large tomatoes, seeded and chopped
- 1 red bell pepper
- 1 cup sun-dried tomatoes
- 1 teaspoon honey
- 1/4 cup extra virgin olive oil
- 2 cloves garlic, crushed
- 3/4 teaspoon sea salt
- pinch of cayenne pepper
- 2 tablespoons minced fresh basil
- 2 tablespoons minced fresh oregano
- 6 medium green zucchini (peeling optional)

DIRECTIONS:

Put all ingredients (except olive oil and zucchini) in food processor and blend to chunky or smooth. Pour into bowl and mix in olive oil.

Transform zucchini into noodles using a spiral slicer.

Toss noodles with enough marinara sauce to coat well and serve immediately.

You can also try making some of these:

Fennel Apple Soup Recipe This fennel apple soup recipe is delicious and nutritious. With only six ingredients, it's easy to make but still full of good flavor.

Basic Hummus Recipe This hummus recipe is the perfect thing to pair with vegetables. It makes for a great snack and is packed full of good fiber. It's also easy and fast to make!

Goat Cheese and Artichoke Dip Recipe — My Goat Cheese and Artichoke Dip Recipe just might convince you to sneak more artichokes into your diet. Perfect as a game-day dip or a mid-day snack.

Cancer-fighting foods

Cancer is recognized worldwide to be a major health problem affecting millions of people each year. More than 1 million people in the United States alone get cancer each year, and as of 2009, a total of 562,340 deaths from cancer were projected to occur in the United States yearly. The good new is there are certain foods — so-called cancer-fighting foods that can help combat cancer.

Cancer is a systemic disease with various causes, some of which include a poor diet, toxin exposure, nutrient deficiencies and to some extent genetics. One extremely important way to prevent and/or treat cancer is nutritionally, through eating a nutrient-dense diet full of cancer-fighting foods and avoiding things that are known to increase cancer risk. But for many people navigating the modern-day food system often seems overwhelming. Ingredients found in ultra-processed foods are being blamed for everything health-related, from cancer and diabetes to reduced kidney function and bone loss. Only adding to the confusion, sometimes even the way we cook otherwise-healthy foods puts them in the cancer-causing foods category while not consuming enough cancer-fighting foods.

Unfortunately, until food manufacturers are forced to clean up the ingredients they use in their products, it's up to us to avoid the worst kinds and to choose cancer-fighting foods. Researchers have known about the dangers associated with some unhealthy habits and cancer-causing foods for decades, while others are just now emerging as possible culprits. Below I outline the association between certain cooking techniques, unhealthy ingredients found in processed foods and the risk for developing cancer.

In order to overcome their disease, many cancer survivors have been fortunate enough to use a combination of natural cancer treatments in conjunction with conventional medical treatments. Today, the early combination of chemotherapy and nutrition therapy is able to save the lives of thousands of cancer patients. This duel approach can help support the entire body and mind in the healing process, which sometimes be long and very difficult. Certainly when it comes to cancer prevention, more research is still needed. But for now, I'll share the types of foods and ingredients I'd recommend avoiding most, plus tips for how to transition to eating an anti-cancer diet full of cancer-fighting foods.

Are You Eating Enough Cancer-Fighting Foods Every Day?

While we often think of the word "cancer" as one type of disease, this term actually encompasses over 100 different cellular disorders in the body. Cancer refers to uncontrolled cell division that leads to a tumor or abnormal cell growth. When abnormal cells divide without control, they can invade nearby tissues and spread to other parts of the body, including the blood and lymphatic systems.

What does work when it comes to lowering inflammation and fighting free radical damage? The key is consuming plenty of cancer-fighting foods with antioxidants and natural anti-inflammatory phytonutrients. This means avoiding packaged and processed foods and focusing on only those that do not contain antibiotics, chemicals or toxins. Buying foods that are organic, grass-fed, pasture-raised and additive-free can greatly lower the toxic load of your diet.

Findings from the 2010 European Prospective Investigation into Cancer and Nutrition (EPIC) that looked at dietary factors associated with higher cancer risks showed that there's significant associations between cancer risk and low intakes of certain nutrients. (2) Data from the investigation that was published in the European Journal of Cancer showed an inverse association between higher intakes of vitamin C, carotenoids, retinol, α-tocopherol and fiber with overall cancer risk.

After following over 519,978 participants living in 10 European nations, results showed that those who most closely followed a style of eating similar to the Mediterranean diet had the most protection against cancer. High intake of cancer-fighting foods like vegetables, fruit, fish, calcium-rich foods and fiber was associated with a decreased risk of colorectal, lung and breast cancers, while red and processed meat intake, alcohol intake, unhealthy body mass index (BMI), and abdominal obesity were associated with an increased risk. Being physically active and obtaining enough vitamin D also helped lower cancer susceptibility.

Meanwhile, a keto diet that eliminates excess refined sugar and other processed carbohydrates may be effective in reducing or fighting cancer. It's not a coincidence that some of the best cancer-fighting foods are on the keto diet food list.

Cancer-Fighting Foods vs. Cancer-Causing Foods

Inflammation is the underlying issue that dictates cancerous tumor initiation, progression and growth. Studies suggest that 30 percent to 40 percent of all kinds of cancer can be prevented with a healthy lifestyle and dietary measures! (3) And other sources claim that this number is in fact much higher, with around 75 percent of cancer cases being lifestyle-related.

Here are examples of some cancer-causing foods you might not realize are in your diet:

1. Processed Meats

While quality meats, fish and dairy products can be included in an anti-cancer diet, processed meats are definitely something to avoid. The American Cancer Society states on their website that "The International

Agency for Research on Cancer (IARC) has classified processed meat as a carcinogen, something that causes cancer. And it has classified red meat as a probable carcinogen, or something that probably causes cancer." A recent meta-analysis of 800 studies found evidence that eating 50 grams of processed meat every day (equal to about 4 strips of bacon or one hot dog) increased the risk of colorectal cancer by 18 percent.

Processed meats are those that have been treated, altered or preserved to improve taste and prolong freshness. They can contain additives such as nitrates and tend to be very high in sodium. A clue that is a meat is processed is if it's been prepared in any of the following ways: salting, curing, smoking. Examples of processed meats include hot dogs, ham, bacon, sausage, and some deli meats/cold-cuts.

2. Fried, Burnt and Overly Cooked Foods

In early 2017, Britain's Food Standards Agency launched a campaign to help people better understand, and to avoid, the toxin called acrylamide. Acrylamide is found in things like cigarette smoke and is also used in industrial processes like making dyes and plastics. What's surprising is that acrylamide is also a chemical that forms on certain foods, especially starchy foods like bread, crackers, cakes and potatoes, when they are cooked for long periods at high temperatures.

The International Agency for Research on Cancer classifies acrylamide as a "probable human carcinogen" based on data showing it can increase the risk of some types of cancer in lab animals. Acrylamide is mainly found in highly-cooked plant foods like potato and grain products, such as French fries, potato chips, and to some extent coffee. The chemical reaction occurs when certain starchy foods are cooked above about 250° F. This causes sugars and the amino acid asparagine to create acrylamide. Note: Acrylamide does not form (or forms at lower levels) in dairy, meat, and fish products.

3. Added Sugar

Sugar can do more than increase your calorie intake and contribute to an expanding waistline— high consumption of added sugar has also been associated with increased cancer risk. There's evidence that added sugars, such as high fructose corn syrup, may increase the risk of esophageal cancer, small intestine cancer, colon cancer and breast cancer. (8, 9, 10) A number of studies have found that sugar not only contributes to problems like obesity and diabetes, but is also linked to increased growth of tumors and metastasis.

Here's another reason to avoid too much sugar: studies have found that people getting 17 to 21 percent of calories from added sugar face a 38 percent higher risk of dying from cardiovascular disease compared to those who got just 8 percent of their calories from sugar.

4. Foods High in Additives

A 2016 study published in Cancer Research discovered a link between common food additives and colon cancer. Researchers at Georgia State University's Institute for Biomedical Sciences found that mice that regularly ingested the dietary emulsifiers called polysorbate-80 and carboxymethylcellulose experienced exacerbated tumor development and increased, low-grade inflammation and colon carcinogenesis.

These emulsifiers act as "detergent-like" ingredients in the gut, significantly changing the species composition of the gut microbiome. Alterations in bacterial species can result in bacteria expressing more flagellins and lipopolysaccharides; in other words, changes in the microbiome can interfere with functions of the immune system, promote inflammation and increase harmful gene expressions. What types of processed foods and products contain these emulsifiers? Examples include dairy products such as ice cream, creamy beauty products, toothpaste, mouthwash, laxatives, diet pills, water-based paints, detergents and even vaccines.

5. Rice Products

Drinking water contaminated with arsenic can increase a person's risk of lung, skin and bladder cancers. That's why there are clear limits set for the amount of arsenic allowed in water. But what about the arsenic present in the food supply? Turns out, most Americans get more arsenic from the foods in their diet than from the water they drink. So is arsenic poisoning from foods like rice something you need to consider?

While babies potentially face the highest risk, excess arsenic isn't good for any of us. A 2012 Consumer Reports investigation found arsenic in every brand of infant rice cereals it tested – nearly ten times the legal limit for drinking water! Subsequent testing was even more dire: just one serving of infant rice cereal can put children over the weekly maximum advised by Consumer Reports.

According to the The Environmental Working Group's (EWG) website, "Heavy metals like arsenic, cadmium and lead are naturally present in water and soil. In some places, intense concentrations exist as a result of industrial pollution and decades of agricultural use of lead- and arsenic-based pesticides." Organizations like the EWG and the World Health Organization now recommend limiting consumption of rice and rice-based foods (including those containing rice flour) when possible and instead eat a varied diet of healthy lower-arsenic grains and sweeteners.

Just like with heart disease, diabetes, leaky gut syndrome and other autoimmune disorders, free radical damage or oxidative stress from inflammation is truly at the root of cancer formation. What does this mean in terms of choosing the very best cancer-fighting foods that you can? Lots of fruit and vegetables can help lower the risk of cancer and offer protective elements so these should be the bases of your diet. On top of that, obtaining enough healthy proteins and fatty acids keeps your immune system working properly and prevents muscle wasting, deficiencies, or hormonal and nerve problems.

Cancer-Fighting Foods

1. Leafy Green Vegetables

Leafy greens are the cornerstone of any healthy diet since they're exceptionally rich in vitamins, minerals, antioxidants and enzymes, yet very low in calories, fats, sodium and other toxins. Leafy greens of all kinds — nutritious spinach, kale, collard greens, romaine, arugula salad, watercress, etc. — are rich in antioxidants known to combat cancer, including vitamin C and beta-carotene (a type of vitamin A).

And the benefits keep coming; as natural sources of glucosinolates, they also contain antibacterial and antiviral properties, inactivate carcinogens, help reprogram cancer cells to die off, and prevent tumor formation and metastasis. These powerhouse chemicals are known to break down during the chewing and digestion process into biologically active compounds that prevent cancer cells growth, which are referred to as indoles, thiocyanates and isothiocyanates.

Isothiocyanates (ITCs) found in leafy greens, which are made from glucosinolates, have been reported to help detox your body at the cellular level. Add a handful of leafy greens to your lunch and dinner to increase your nutrient intake; to make obtaining them simpler, try juicing vegetables for near perfect health. Vegetable juices are very easy to digest and make yourself at home. The Gerson diet meal plan even advises cancer patients to drink 13 glasses of freshly prepared juice daily!

2. Cruciferous Vegetables

Cruciferous vegetables are known to be powerful cancer killers and some of the best vitamin C foods widely available. Many are rich in glutathione, known as the body's "master antioxidant" since it has high free-radical-scavenging abilities. Nearly all members of the brassica family of cruciferous vegetables are nutrient-dense sources of a family of phytochemicals called isothiocyanates that are linked to cancer prevention. In addition to isothiocyanates, cruciferous veggies like cabbage and broccoli also contain sulforaphanes and indoles — two types of strong antioxidants and stimulators of detoxifying enzymes that protect the structure of DNA.

Add one or two kinds — including broccoli, cauliflower, cabbage or Brussels sprouts — to three mostly plant-based meals daily in the form of roasted veggies, soups or stir fries, or dip them into hummus or Greek yogurt for a healthy, fast snack. Additionally, many other vegetables are beneficial for lowering cancer risk, including onions, zucchini, asparagus, artichokes, peppers, carrots and beets.

3. Berries

The ORAC scores of nearly all berries are very high, making them some of the top high-antioxidant foods in the world. Blueberries, raspberries, cherries, strawberries, goji berries, camu camu and blackberries are easy to find and use in numerous types of recipes — which is good news considering they supply vitamin C, vitamin A and gallic acid, a powerful antifungal/antiviral agent that increases immunity.

Berries are especially rich in proanthocyanidin antioxidants, which have been observed to have anti-aging properties in several animal studies and are capable of lowering free radical damage. High amounts of phenols, zeaxanthin, lycopene, cryptoxanthin, lutein and polysaccharides are other berry benefits. Less familiar "superfoods" mulberry, camu camu and goji berries have been used in traditional Chinese medicine since around 200 B.C. to increase immunity and energy, so look for those in powder or dried form in health food stores and online.

4. Brightly Orange-Colored Fruits and Veggies (Citrus Fruits, Squash, Sweet Potatoes, etc.)

Brightly colored pigments found in plant foods are a sure sign that they're beaming with phytochemicals, especially carotenoid antioxidants. This is exactly the reason you want to "eat the rainbow" and vary the colors of the foods on your plate.

Carotenoids (alpha-carotene, beta-carotene, lycopene, lutein, cryptoxanthin) are derivatives of vitamin A found in many citrus fruits, sweet potatoes, berries, pumpkin, squashes and other plant foods. (14) One of the most researched is beta-carotene, an essential nutrient for immune functioning; detoxification; liver health; and fighting cancers of the skin, eyes and organs. Two nutrients that give these foods their signature dark hues include lutein and zeaxanthin, which have been shown to help prevent eye and skin-related disorders since they act as antioxidants that filter harmful high-energy blue wavelengths, protecting healthy cells in the process.

When it comes to carbohydrate-rich veggies, studies show that complex carbs, including sweet potatoes, carrots, beets, other tubers and whole-grain foods, is related to a reduced risk of several types of cancer, particularly of the upper digestive tract. This is likely due to a favorable role of fiber, but the issue is still open to discussion. In contrast, refined grain intake and high glycemic load foods are not apart of an anti-cancer diet. These have been associated with increased risk of different types of cancer, including breast and colorectal. (15)

5. Fresh Herbs and Spices

Turmeric, which contains the active ingredient curcumin, is one of the most powerful ingredients in an anti-cancer diet because it's been shown to decrease tumor size and fight colon and breast cancer. Along with easy-to-use black pepper, turmeric absorption is enhanced and better able to fight inflammation. Aim for one teaspoon of turmeric powder and 1/4 teaspoon of black pepper or more daily, which can easily be used in a tonic drink, with eggs or in a veggie stir fry. You can also take curcumin supplements; aim for 1,000 milligrams daily.

Additionally, other herbs that act as immune system boosters include ginger, raw garlic, thyme, cayenne pepper, oregano, basil and parsley which can easily be used in many recipes, juices, dressings and smoothies.

6. Organic Meats

Organic meats including beef or chicken liver are recommended on many cancer-fighting diets since they're considered some of the most nutrient-dense foods on the planet and extremely high in vitamin B12. Consuming organic meats as part of a "nose to tail" approach to eating animal proteins provides minerals that help cleanse the liver and enhance the ability to remove toxins from the blood and digestive tract.

Detoxifying with rich sources of selenium, zinc and B vitamins helps purify blood; produce the bile needed to digest fats; balance hormones naturally; and store essential vitamins, minerals and iron. These mineral-rich foods can help counteract the effects of alcohol, prescription drugs, hormone disruptions, high triglyceride levels, low potassium, obesity and viral infections.

7. Cultured Dairy Products

Cultured dairy products are a rich source of "good bacteria" probiotics, which are microorganisms that promote a natural bacterial balance in your intestinal microflora and help increase immunity. Over 80 percent of your immune system is housed in your gut, so it's no surprise that probiotic foods and supplementation can stop tumor growth and help cells renew.

One of the easiest ways to consume more probiotics is in their most natural state, which includes raw milk products such as cheese, kefir and yogurt. Raw and cultured are key here, since fermentation produces probiotics but high heat processing used to pasteurize dairy can damage many of the vital nutrients, including the enzymes, proteins and probiotics. Most dairy today is loaded with hormones, antibiotics, pain killers and pesticide residue so buying organic is also important.

Aim for six ounces of cultured dairy daily (probiotic yogurt, cottage cheese, goat milk kefir or amasai). Cottage cheese, which is rich in sulfur protein and saturated fats, was found to be especially beneficial as part of the Budwig diet for cancer protocol. You can also increase your probiotic food intake without dairy by consuming cultured vegetables like kimchi, sauerkraut, coconut kefir, kombucha or natto.

Cultured dairy is also a great source of calcium. Calcium, particularly when combined with Vitamin D3 form, may reduce the incidence of cancer by 35 to 60 percent. Calcium seems to be especially beneficial for preventing cancer and rectal cancers. (16) Some studies have also found that it helps reduce breast cancer and ovarian cancer risk. Sunlight exposure and marine oils such as cod liver oil or krill oil are great sources of vitamin D that help with calcium absorption. Calcium should ideally be obtained from foods like organic dairy products (I recommend

8. Nuts and Seeds

Chia seeds and flaxseeds are two of the most nutrient-dense seeds in the world. They provide fiber, omega-3 fatty acids and a range of important minerals. Hemp seeds, sesame seeds, pumpkin seeds and sunflower seeds are also beneficial and full of healthy fatty acids, as are walnuts, brazil nuts and almonds. Their health benefits and are best sprouted and can be used easily in smoothies, baked goods and with yogurt. Aim for two tablespoons daily.

9. Healthy Unrefined Oils (Coconut, Flax, Cod Liver and Extra Virgin Olive Oil)

Did you know that your brain and nervous system control the function of your entire body and that about 60 percent of your nervous system is made up of fatty acids? The problem is that many of the conventional processed fats and oils widely consumed today are hydrogenated oils that are capable of destroying the membranes of our cells, leading to diseased cells and toxicity.

Refined and rancid fats create problems throughout your entire body, leading to lower immune function, cell congestion and inflammation that kicks off disease.

Replace refined vegetable oils, hydrogenated oils and trans fats with quality oils, including flax oil, extra virgin olive oil, cod oil and coconut oil. These nourish your gut and promote better immune function, help you reach and maintain a healthy weight, plus flaxseed and cod liver oil contain essential omega-3 fatty acids that can help energize your cells. Olive oil contains phytonutrients that seem to reduce inflammation in the body. It may reduce the risk of breast and colorectal cancers.

10. Mushrooms

Nutritious mushrooms vary in terms of their benefits, taste and appearance since hundreds of mushroom species are in existence today, but all are known to be immune-enhancers and many have been used to fight cancer for centuries.(17) Reishi, cordyceps and maitake in particular can improve immune function, fight tumor growth and help with cell regeneration. Look for them in capsule or tincture form, and cook with them whole whenever possible too.

11. Traditional Teas

Metastasis is the most deadly aspect of cancer and results from several connected processes including cell proliferation, angiogenesis, cell adhesion, migration and invasion into the surrounding tissue. Metastasis is the principal cause of death among cancer patients, so it's one of the most important issues in cancer research today. Several clinical and epidemiological studies have reported that the consumption of green tea can help decrease cancer risk. Green tea contains major polyphenolic compounds, including epigallocatechin-3-gallate, which has been shown to inhibit tumor invasion and angiogenesis, which are essential for tumor growth and metastasis.

Teas derived from the leaves of the plant Camellia sinensis are commonly consumed as beverages around the world, including green, black or oolong tea. While all traditional teas seem to be beneficial, the most significant effects on human health have been attributed to green tea, such as matcha green tea. It contains the highest percetange of polyphenolic compounds, catechin, gallocatechin and EGCG.

The antioxidant EGCG appears to be the most potent of all the catechins, and its anticancer effects have activity about 25–100 times more effective than that of vitamins C and E! EGCG has been reported to be linked to the modulation of multiple signaling pathways, finally resulting in the downregulation of expression of proteins involved in the invasiveness of cancer cells.

12. Wild-Caught Fish

According to a 2004 study conducted by researchers at the Richerche Institute of Pharmacology, higher fish consumption is another favorable diet indicator of better immune function.the study, which investigated the cancer-fighting effects of the Mediterranean diet, found that people who reported eating less fish and more frequent red meat showed several common neoplasms in their blood that suggested higher susceptibility.

Wild and especially small fish, including salmon, mackerel and sardines are anti-inflammatory omega-3 foods that are correlated with better brain, hormonal and nervous system health. Omega-3 fatty acids exert anti-inflammatory effects, and therefore recent studies have connected them to cancer prevention and natural enhancement of antitumour therapies. Evidence suggests a role for omega-3 fatty acid supplementation in cancer prevention and reducing symptoms of treatments like chemotherapy. Omega-3s have been shown to preserve muscle mass and function in chemotherapy cancer patients and to contribute to a reduced inflammatory response resulting from the treatment's toxicity.

Other Ways to Increase Effectiveness of An Anti-Cancer Diet

1. Lower Your Toxin Load

An anti-cancer diet consists of:

Lowering your toxin intake.

Supporting the body's cleansing and detoxifying processes.

Eating healthy and nutrient-rich foods to support all of your body's functions.

First and foremost, you can take these steps to reduce or eliminate the following products and substances from your life in order to halt toxin accumulation and reduce free radical, cellular damage:

Electromagnetic Waves: Cell phones, TV's, computer screens, microwaves—even the wiring in our homes and basic appliances emit constant electromagnetic frequencies or EMF's that disturb the bioelectrical functioning of our bodies. Cell phone use has been linked to a host of cancer-promoting processes. Limit your exposure by getting rid of your microwave, as it is your largest source for EMF's, and making use of headphones with your cell phone.

Commercial Health and Beauty Products: The things we put in our mouths and use on our skin or hair, such as commercial shampoos, makeup and cleansing products, are often loaded with potential carcinogens. Visit the Environmental Working Group's SkinDeep database to look-up your favorite products and determine if you should switch to another brand.

Household Cleaners: Indoor environments are often concentrated sources of pollution. Lower your toxin load by switching to natural cleaners or making your own instead of using products that are filled with chemicals.

Unnecessary Medications: All medications pass through and burden the liver. High use of acetaminophen is rapidly overtaking alcohol as the number one cause of liver disease. Work with your physician to lessen the amount of medications you are taking.

Plastics: Compounds in plastic containers, plastic wraps, the lining of metal cans, and paperboard containers can all leach compounds that disrupt the neuroendocrine system. This is especially true when plastic is heated, which is why it's smart not to microwave plastic containers, store very hot food in plastic, or leave plastic water bottles anywhere where they will become very hot (such as in your car).

You may also want to periodically try fasting to help with detoxification. Even if you eat healthy foods regularly, environmental toxins bombard you at all turns. The organs that are responsible for detoxification and elimination–the skin, respiratory system, kidney, liver and digestive tractoften get overburdened and re-circulate toxins in the bloodstream. Practicing a cleanse or detox every few months can help these organs "catch up" and dispose of toxins stored in cells and tissue. Colon and liver cleanses can be accomplished with a variety of herbs, green drinks and easily digested whole foods such as juiced vegetables or those that are lightly steamed.

2. Drink Clean Water

Our drinking (tap) water can contain hundreds of unregulated substances, from pesticides and heavy metals to hormones and other pollutants. Bottled water is even less regulated, which means it's not necessarily a good alternative. Your best bet is buying a filter that can be used as home to remove chlorine, fluoride and other pollutants from the water you drink and cook with.

3. Cook Foods at Lower Temperatures and Avoid Burnt Food

Don't fry your foods! Greatly reduce the amount of fast food, french fries, chips, cakes, cereals and crackers you eat.

It's virtually impossible to completely eliminate acrylamide that can accumulate on fried foods. But eating a balanced diet mostly free of processed foods and avoiding a high-starch diet can greatly reduce acrylamide levels.

Frying, baking, broiling or roasting are more likely to create acrylamide. On the other hand, boiling and steaming appear less likely to do so. Longer cooking times and cooking at higher temperatures can increase the amount of acrylamide in foods further.

Don't store potatoes in the refrigerator. That can cause acrylamide levels to surge. If you're planning on cooking potatoes at higher temperatures, soak the cut-up spuds first. Soaking in water for 2 hours before high-temp cooking can reduce acrylamide levels by nearly 50 percent. Even a simple 30-second rinse can slash acrylamide levels by 20-plus percent.

I don't eat much bread, but when I do eat an occasional sandwich or toast, I make sure it's made with sprouted bread, such as Ezekiel bread. Additionally, I definitely avoid over-toasting or burning the bread! The Food Standards Agency says as a general rule of thumb, aim for a golden yellow color or lighter when toasting, roasting, frying or baking.

4. Avoid Processed Grains and Added Sugar

Our bodies make best use of food in its natural state, which is why added sugar or processed/refined grains are difficult to break down and can cause gut trouble. The more processed and altered that a food is, the more unnatural and harmful it becomes. Refined sugar, wheat flour, boxed pastas, frozen dinners, powdered cheese and heat-treated vegetable oils these processed foods are at the heart of a whole host of diseases and disorders.

Wheat, soy and corn products are highly subsidized by the US government, making them very cheap and widely available for production of highly processed and refined products. Food allergies associated with these foods are subsequently on the rise and can contribute to leaky gut syndrome and improper nutrient absorption. These foods are also often loaded with pesticides, herbicides, GMOs and heavy metals. More and more, the seeds from which they are grown are genetically engineered. The solution? Buy organic, sprouted whole grains and avoid processed soy products.

Check ingredient labels to be sure you're not consuming high amounts of added sugar/sweeteners. Brown rice syrup found in some snack bars and non-dairy beverages may contain high arsenic levels.

Be wary of foods that might seem healthy but are really not, such as low-fat or fat-free foods, dairy-free and gluten-free foods, rice milk and foods containing artificial sweeteners. Many times these foods contain chemical additives in order to replace fat, wheat or dairy ingredients.

Try working alternative grains like quinoa or buckwheat into some meals, rather than eating lots of bread, instant rice, pasta, cereal, etc.

Rinse, soak and sprout your grains. Rinse your rice and cook it like pasta to reduce the amount of antinutrients it will provide. According to a Cornell University researcher, rinsing brown rice until the water is clear (usually 5 to 6 washings), and then cooking in a ration of 1 cup of rice to 6 cups of water, can remove 40 to 55 percent of inorganic arsenic in rice. (22, 23) And researchers from the UK found that cooking rice in a coffee pot reduced arsenic by up to 85 percent.

Consumer Reports testing found that basmati rice grown in California contained the lowest levels of arsenic; all types of rice, except sushi and quick-cooking rice, from Texas, Louisiana, and Arkansas contained the highest levels of inorganic arsenic in a Consumer Reports testing.

5. Use Essential Oils

Frankincense essential oil (Boswellia serrata) has been clinically shown to be a vital treatment for various forms of cancer, including breast, brain, colon and prostate cancers. Frankincense has the ability to help regulate cellular epigenetic function, which positively influences genes to promote healing. Rub frankincense essential oil on your body (neck area) three times daily and take three drops internally in eight ounces of water three times daily as part of a natural prevention plan. Other helpful anti-inflammatory essential oils include clove, rose, tea tree and oregano oils.

6. Get Enough Sunshine and Vitamin D

Vitamin D is a fat-soluble vitamin that acts similarly to a hormone in our bodies. The best way to naturally obtain enough is through direct exposure to the sun, although eating certain vitamin D-rich foods like salmon and eggs can help, as can taking a high-quality supplement.

Clinical research shows that vitamin D can help prevent cancer best when you acquire about 50–70 nanograms per milliliter daily.Cover your bases of vitamin D3 through getting 20 minutes of sun exposure every day, ideally between 10 a.m. and 2 p.m. with 40 percent of your entire body exposed to the sun. You can also take an oral supplement containing around 5,000 to 10,000 IUs of D3 every day; I recommend an effective combination formula of astaxanthin and omega-3 fish oils with vitamin D3 taken together.

7. Boost Detoxification with Supplements and Herbs

Some experts recommend drinking alkaline water which you can create by adding lemon or lime juice and/or a few drops of hydrogen peroxide.To help with detoxification you may also want to increase your intake of raw foods and green juices. Although fiber is an important part of digestion, elimination, detoxification and a source of probiotic support—too much fiber can stress a weakened or hyper-reactive immune system. Juicing, steaming and lightly cooking raw foods, using green powders and cutting back on or eliminating whole grains can ease digestion and make many nutrients more readily available.

Eating a healthy diet is number one when it comes to cancer prevention. But there are also certain herbs and supplements that have been shown to help lower inflammation, boost the immune system, and therefore help to decrease cancer risk. These include:

Alpha-linolenic acid (Omega-3 fatty acid): Omega-3 fatty acids are getting so much attention because the Western diet is so unbalanced with an overabundance of omega-6's. Omega-3's have a host of health benefits and research is still underway to validate their benefits in combating cancer.

Chorella, Blue-green algae and Spirulina: These single-celled animals are a source of Vitamin B12 and bind with heavy metals, helping to eliminate them from the body.

CLA: Conjugated linoleic acid boosts the immune system and may reduce the risk of developing colon, rectal and breast cancers.

Coriolus Mushrooms: These disease fighting mushrooms have specific polysaccharides that boost the immune system, reduce tumor growth and combat cancer.

Folate/Vitamin B9: Folate (vitamin B9) is crucial to DNA production and has been found to be effective against breast, colorectal and pancreatic cancers.

Melatonin: Melatonin is a hormone that helps to regulate our sleep and waking cycles. This hormone's levels are closely linked to immune system function. Getting at least 8 hours of sleep and reducing stress will boost your melatonin levels.

Cancer-Fighting Foods Recipes

The No. 1 thing to do immediately to protect yourself from cancer is to improve your diet. Focus on filling your plate with nutrient-dense vegetables first, and then add in all of the other components that make up a healthy diet. Here's some recipes to get you started:

Anti-Inflammatory Juice Recipe

Pumpkin Blueberry Pancakes Recipe

Kale Chips Recipe

Gluten-Free Cauliflower Mac and Cheese Recipe

Teriyaki Baked Salmon Recipe

Precautions Regarding An Anti-Cancer Diet and Cancer-Fighting Foods

The quality of your diet is undoubtably linked to your overall health and ability to prevent cancer. However other factors are also important for cancer-prevention, such as exercising, avoiding medication and toxin exposure, not smoking or consuming too much alcohol, sleeping well and controlling stress. A variety of foods can be included in an anti-cancer diet, and your diet doesn't need to be "perfect" to be healthy. Start by making one or two changes at a time to your diet, removing foods that you consume a lot of but that are known to increase cancer risk.

Final Thoughts on Cancer-Fighting Foods

Cancer-causing foods, as opposed to cancer-fighting foods, include those that contain pesticides, additives, added sugar or artificial sweeteners, processed meats, burnt foods, fried foods and other chemicals. Examples of cancer-causing foods and ingredients are french fries, hot dogs, deli meats, sausage, ice cream, refined rice and other gains, high fructose corn syrup, processed vegetable oils, and trans-fats.

To follow an anti-cancer diet, lower your toxin intake, support the body's cleansing and detoxifying processes, get enough vitamin D, upgrade your water and eat unprocessed nutrient-rich foods — in addition to cancer-fighting foods.

Some of the top cancer-fighting foods include cruciferous veggies, leafy greens, berries, orange and yellow veggies, herbs and spices, cultured dairy products, nuts, seeds and healthy fats like coconut or olive oil.

Mediterranean diet for cancer

Evidence research

Cancer prevention

Overall incidence of cancer is lower in Mediterranean countries compared to the United States, United Kingdom, and the Scandinavian countries.2 Large prospective observational studies have linked the Mediterranean diet to this decreased cancer incidence. For example, the MOLI-SANI Project transformed the Molise region of Italy into a "scientific laboratory" of data collection, specifically looking at cardiovascular disease and cancer in relationship to the Mediterranean diet. Other large observational studies, such as the European Prospective Investigation into Cancer and Nutrition (EPIC) and the National Institutes of Health-American Association for Retired Persons (NIH-AARP) Diet and Health study, have subanalyzed the data, looking at the Mediterranean diet, cancer markers, incidence, and mortality. The Greek cohort of the EPIC study (N=25,623) was followed for 7.9 years. Investigators found a 12% reduction in cancer incidence for every 2-point increase in the 10-point Mediterranean diet adherence scale.3 The NIH-AARP Diet and Health study (N=380,296) found a 17% and 12% decreased cancer mortality in men and women following the Mediterranean diet after 5 years of follow-up.4

Breast cancer

Several clinical trials have built upon the data from prospective observational studies. The PREvención con DIeta MEDiterránea (PREDIMED) study is the most well-known, and many analyses have been published from the PREDIMED data. This parallel-group, randomized, multicenter, controlled 5-year trial originally aimed to assess the effects of the Mediterranean diet in primary prevention of cardiovascular disease. A total of 7,447 participants, including 4,282 who were at high risk of cardiovascular events, were randomized to follow one of the following 3 diets: low-fat diet; Mediterranean diet with added EVOO; or Mediterranean diet with added nuts. When compared to a low-fat diet, the risk of combined heart attack, stroke, and death from cardiovascular disease was reduced by 30% in Mediterranean diet + EVOO group and 28% in Mediterranean diet + nuts group.

Cardiovascular risk factors such as blood glucose, blood pressure, low-density lipoprotein (LDL)-cholesterol and C-reactive protein (CRP) were all reduced,5 and the risk of developing type 2 diabetes fell by 52%.6 As an added bonus, in the female cohort they discovered a 68% reduced risk of developing breast cancer in the Mediterranean diet + EVOO group when compared to the low-fat diet group. Each additional 5% of calories from EVOO yielded a hazard ratio of 0.72. An overall 51% reduced risk of breast cancer incidence was found for both Mediterranean diet groups combined. The authors concluded that "this is the first randomized trial finding an effect of a long-term dietary intervention on breast cancer incidence."7

The NIH-AARP Diet and Health study (N=380,296) found a 17% and 12% decreased cancer mortality in men and women following the Mediterranean diet after 5 years of follow-up.

Now let us look at secondary prevention of breast cancer. Preliminary results of the "SETA PROJECT" were released at the 2016 American Society of Clinical Oncology (ASCO) annual meeting. Of 307 women treated for early-stage breast cancer, 199 were assigned to follow a "normal diet with dietary advice to reduce the occurrence of cancer relapse" (referred to as the Std-Diet) and 109 were assigned to follow the Mediterranean diet. After 3 years of follow-up, 11 cases of recurrence were discovered in the Std-Diet group and no recurrence was found in the Mediterranean diet group.8 Statistical significance was achieved; however, this study is ongoing and we look forward to additional data. Further studies are needed to better evaluate the effect of the Mediterranean diet on secondary prevention such as the DIANA (Diet and Androgens)-5 study that is evaluating the effects of a Mediterranean-macrobiotic diet in women diagnosed with early-stage invasive breast cancer.

Of note, there is a particular benefit from the Mediterranean diet in the incidence of double- and triple-negative breast cancers. Subanalysis of data from the Grupo Español de Investigación en Cáncer de Mama (EpiGEICAM) study shows a 44% reduced risk of all breast cancer incidence and a 68% reduced risk of development of triple-negative tumors when comparing top vs bottom quartile of Mediterranean diet adherence.10 Data from the EPIC study shows a 7% reduced risk of postmenopausal breast cancer incidence and a 20% reduced risk of estrogen receptor-negative/progesterone receptor-negative breast cancer in high vs low Mediterranean diet adherence.

Colorectal cancer

The Mediterranean diet is also associated with a reduced risk of colorectal cancer incidence. The Adventist Health Study 2, a prospective North American cohort trial of 77,659 Seventh-day Adventist men and women, compared 4 vegetarian dietary patterns—vegan, lacto-ovo vegetarian, pescovegetarian, and semivegetarian—to a nonvegetarian diet. After 7.3 years of follow-up, the pescovegetarian cohort showed a 43% reduced risk of colorectal cancer incidence when compared with nonvegetarians.12 The Mediterranean diet can be described as primarily pescovegetarian. Data from the EPIC study shows 8% or 11% reduced risk of colorectal cancer incidence,13 depending on the type of Mediterranean diet assessment used, and a 46% reduced risk specifically in the Italian cohort.14 A meta-analysis of 4 prospective cohort and 4 case-control studies of Mediterranean diet and colorectal cancer showed an overall 17% risk reduction.

Other cancer types

The Mediterranean diet has shown benefit for a reduced risk of many other cancer types. Data from the EPIC study shows a 33% reduced risk of gastric cancer incidence while a meta-analysis shows a 27% reduced risk. A 42% reduced risk of liver cancer incidence was found in 2 studies. The NIH-AARP Diet and Health study showed a 56% reduced risk of squamous cell carcinoma of the esophagus.15

Mechanisms of Action

Metabolic syndrome

Growing data support the association of metabolic syndrome and its components with cancer development and cancer-related mortality. A systemic review and meta-analysis shows a strong link between cancer and metabolic syndrome, with a 61% increased incidence for endometrial, 58% for pancreatic, 56% for postmenopausal breast, and 52% for rectal cancers in women with metabolic syndrome.

An intervention study of 180 participants with metabolic syndrome were equally divided to follow the Mediterranean diet or the Prudent diet (control). After 2 years of follow-up, resolution of metabolic syndrome was seen in 50 vs 12 patients, respectively. Compared to controls, those following the Mediterranean diet increased their intake of monounsaturated fat, polyunsaturated fat, fiber, fruit, vegetables, nuts, whole grains, and olive oil, with a lower ratio of omega-6/3. The Mediterranean diet group had significantly reduced hs-CRP, interleukin (IL)-7, IL-18, and insulin resistance, and improved endothelial function.

Data from the PREDIMED trial showed a 35% increased resolution of metabolic syndrome in the Mediterranean diet with EVOO group and 28% in the Mediterranean diet with nuts group when compared to the control diet group. They found significant decreases in central obesity and high fasting glucose. They concluded that "the abundance of healthy, nutrient-dense foods that make up the plant-based Mediterranean diet predicts its bioactivity and potential to beneficially influence metabolic pathways that lead to MetS [metabolic syndrome] and T2 DM [type 2 diabetes mellitus] as well as other chronic conditions."

Weight loss

Extra adipose tissue can have deleterious effects on the body that affect the metabolic milieu and raise the risk of cancer incidence and progression, such as producing hormone and growth factors and increasing inflammatory markers. For many of our patients seeking primary and secondary cancer prevention, achieving a healthy weight is an important goal. The PREDIMED study did not restrict calories or encourage physical activity, yet a 0.43 kg weight loss was found in the Mediterranean diet with EVOO group and a 0.94 cm decreased waist circumference was found in the Mediterranean diet with nuts group.19 In an intervention trial comparing low-fat, Mediterranean, and low-carbohydrate diets in 322 moderately obese participants, the Mediterranean diet group lost 4.4 kg, compared to 2.9 kg in the low-fat group, and 4.7 kg in the low-carbohydrate group after 2 years of follow-up.20

Inflammation

Inflammation is recognized as a major factor in the pathology of many chronic diseases, including cardiovascular disease, diabetes mellitus, Alzheimer's disease, and, of course, cancer. Diet plays an important role in either increasing or decreasing the inflammatory response, depending on dietary choices. Acute inflammation can occur during the postprandial state as a result of hyperlipidemia and hyperglycemia. This can be exacerbated by advanced glycation end products (AGEs) and mitigated by antioxidants in the diet. Healthy dietary patterns are associated with lower circulating concentrations of inflammatory markers. Whole grains, vegetables, fruits, and fish, all important components of the Mediterranean diet, are all associated with lower inflammation.

A 2010 systematic literature review found that the Mediterranean diet is associated with lower circulating markers of inflammation.The MOLI-SANI study evaluated for low-grade inflammation based on CRP, leukocyte, platelet counts, and granulocyte/lymphocyte ratio, and decreased levels of these inflammatory markers were detected in relation to the Mediterranean diet. The granulocyte/lymphocyte ratio is of particular interest as it is not only a marker of inflammation, but is also associated with a poorer prognosis in cancer acting as an independent predictor of tumor growth, metastasis, and progression.23

Antioxidant action

Free radical damage can have direct effects on DNA. Regular consumption of antioxidants in the diet improves total antioxidant capacity, thereby protecting the cell. Oxidative damage can also have secondary effects by increasing the inflammatory response and affecting genetic expression. In an extensive review of the link between oxidative stress, inflammation, and cancer, the authors conclude that "oxidative stress can activate NF-κB [nuclear factor kappa light chain enhancer of activated B cells], AP-1, p53, HIF-1α [hypoxia-inducible factor 1-alpha], PPAR-γ [peroxisome proliferator-activated receptor gamma], β-catenin/Wnt, and Nrf2 leading to expression of over 500 different genes, including growth factors, inflammatory cytokines, chemokines, cell cycle regulatory molecules, and anti-inflammatory molecules leading to transformation of a normal cell to tumor cell, tumor cell survival, proliferation, chemoresistance, radioresistance, invasion, angiogenesis and stem cell survival."24

The Mediterranean diet is abundant in antioxidant-rich fruits and vegetables and is linked to increased total antioxidant capacity and decreased oxidative load. Data from the PREDIMED study shows that blood levels of Ferric Reducing Antioxidant Potential (FRAP) at baseline and after 1 year of dietary interventions showed increases in both the Mediterranean diet with EVOO group (FRAP 72.0 µmol/L) and the Mediterranean diet with nuts (48.9 µmol/L) group, but not with the low-fat diet group. Similar results were found for total radical-trapping antioxidant parameters (TRAPs).25 PREDIMED data also found decreased in vivo LDL oxidation in both Mediterranean diet groups.26

Data shows a link between increased antioxidant intake, specifically from the polyphenol content of the Mediterranean diet, and decreases in low-grade inflammation. Polyphenol content of the Mediterranean diet was negatively associated with low-grade inflammation based on decreased levels of CRP, leukocyte, platelet counts, and granulocyte/lymphocyte ratios,27 as well as decreased VCAM-1 and ICAM-1 (cell adhesion molecules), IL-6, tumor necrosis factor (TNF)-α and monocyte chemoattractant protein(MCP) -1.28

Mediterranean Anti-Cancer Recipes

3.5oz/100g firm tofu, sliced and marinated overnight in 2 tbsp basil pesto

3-4 firm tomatoes

1 ripe but firm avocado

2oz/50 g pine nuts olive oil

1 tbsp balsamic vinegar

15 basil leaves, roughly torn or shredded salt & freshly ground black pepper

Avocado, tomato and tofu tricolora salad

Inspired by Italy's insalata tricolora, (tomatoes, mozzarella and basil) this light hors d'oeuvre brims with summer aromas: spicy tomatoes, sweet basil, fruity olive oil, fragrant balsamic vinegar and nutty pine nuts. The innovation is tofu instead of mozzarella. Serves 4.

Slice tofu into ¼-inch/5mm slices and place in a container with a lid. Add pesto (perhaps diluted with a little water to make it runnier) and combine, ensuring that the tofu is well coated with the pesto. Seal and refrigerate for several hours, or ideally overnight.

When you are ready to prepare the salad, slice the tomatoes with a sharp knife, taking care to remove the fibrous core.

Halve the avocado, remove the stone, halve again, peel quarters carefully and slice.

In a dry pan on low heat, toast pine nuts until golden and fragrant (2-3 minutes). Transfer to a bowl to cool.

Arrange tomatoes, avocado and marinated tofu on a large serving plate. Drizzle with olive oil and balsamic vinegar, scatter with pine nuts and basil leaves and season lightly with salt and freshly ground black pepper. Serve immediately.

½ red cabbage, quartered, cored and finely sliced by hand or food processor

1 large apple (peeled if non-organic), finely grated

1 shallot, finely chopped

2 tbsp apple cider or red wine vinegar

2 tbsp raisins

2oz/50g walnuts, coarsely chopped

2 tbsp walnut oil

2 tbsp olive oil salt, pepper

Red cabbage and walnut slaw

A crunchy, fruity and dramatically colored salad for those dreary winter months – this makes a pleasant (and lighter) change from traditional coleslaw with mayonnaise!

In a salad bowl, combine chopped shallot and vinegar and leave to infuse five minutes. Then add oil, salt and pepper.

Add shredded cabbage, grated apple and raisins and toss with dressing; if you have time, leave to infuse for ½ hour. Sprinkle with walnuts and serve.

3 tbsp olive oil

1.1lb/500g chicken leg

portions

2 large onions, chopped

1 rib celery, cubed

1 tbsp freshly grated or dried, ground ginger

3 cloves garlic

1 tsp turmeric

1 tsp ground coriander

½ tsp ground cumin

½ tsp paprika powder pinch of saffron

1 cinnamon stick pinch of chili powder

7oz/200g cubed pumpkin or carrots

15oz/400g cooked garbanzos, drained

15oz/400g cubed tomatoes (fresh or from a jar)

2 pints/1l chicken stock zest and juice of ½ lemon

3 tbsp chopped cilantro salt & freshly ground black pepper

Moroccan chicken & garbanzo soup

This well-known dish (called chorba in Arabic) is a nourishing North African stew often eaten just before sunrise during Ramadan, the Islamic month of fasting. As with so many

Mediterranean stews, there are as many versions of chorba as there are cooks – some prepared with lamb, others with veal, some containing vermicelli noodles, others potatoes. Feel free to add other vegetables such as green beans, chopped fresh spinach, turnips or zucchini, depending on the season and on your mood. However, the garbanzos should remain as they give the soup bulk and bite; if you like, you can replace the chicken with small cubes of firm tofu. Serves 4.

In a large, heavy cooking pot, warm 1 tablespoon olive oil and cook the chicken portions on gentle heat until golden on both sides. Remove and set aside.

Add remaining olive oil and cook onion, celery and garlic until the onions are translucent. Add ginger and spices and cook for another minute, stirring to prevent the spices burning. Add stock and carrots or pumpkin, and bring to a boil.

Return chicken portions to the pot, add garbanzos and bring back to the boil; then reduce heat and simmer on low heat for 20 minutes. Add tomatoes and continue cooking for 15-20 minutes, until the vegetables are soft and the chicken is cooked through.

Remove chicken, discard skin, shred into bite-sized pieces and return to stew to reheat.

Season to taste with lemon zest and juice, salt and pepper and sprinkle with chopped cilantro leaves.

1 large cucumber, cubed

7oz/200g plain yogurt

2oz/50g ground almonds

1 small apple, peeled, cored and cubed

1 clove garlic, crushed

½ bunch of mint (about 5-6 stalks) zest and juice of ½ lemon

3 tbsp olive oil salt & freshly ground black pepper

2 tbsp almond slivers pinch red pepper flakes or paprika powder

Chilled minty cucumber soup

On a hot summer's day, the mere thought of this pale-green, minty concoction will send cool waves through you.

What's more, you won't work up a sweat making it as it is ready in a matter of minutes and there is next-to-no cooking involved!

Serves 4.

In a dry skillet and on low heat, lightly toast almond slivers for

1-2 minutes until barely golden. Transfer to a plate to cool.

Pick the mint leaves off the stalks, set a few aside for garnish and place the rest in a blender along with yogurt, cucumber, lemon juice and zest, almonds, crushed garlic and apple. Blend until smooth and light green. Adjust seasoning to taste. Chill for at least 1 hour; this allows the flavors to deepen.

Serve in individual bowls or glasses decorated with mint leaves. Sprinkle lightly with pepper flakes or paprika powder and toasted almond slivers. For extra cooling effect, add 1-2 ice cubes per glass.

Variation

You can replace the mint with dill and garnish the soup with a teaspoonful of pink salmon roe for a Scandinavian touch.

15oz/400g cherry tomatoes, washed and patted dry

12fl oz/1½ cups/350ml unsweetened almond or soy milk

7oz/200g feta cheese, crumbled

4 eggs large pinch of turmeric (to taste)

2 tbsp corn starch

2 tbsp chopped chives or basil leaves salt & freshly ground black pepper some olive oil for the pie dish

Cherry tomato pie

Clafoutis, a classic French dish, is most widely known in its original incarnation as a sweet cherry pie. This savory version makes a quick and easy summer lunch when tomatoes are sweet and aromatic, and juicy herbs abound. Tastes great with Warm Puy lentil salad or with a lightly tossed green salad. Serves 4.

Preheat oven to 350°F/180°C.

Oil oven-proof ceramic dish and place cherry tomatoes and crumbled feta cheese in it.

In a bowl, whisk corn starch with milk and eggs. Add half the chopped herbs and turmeric and combine into a smooth, creamy batter. Season with salt and pepper.

Pour egg mixture gently over tomatoes and feta cheese and slide the pie dish into the oven. Bake for approximately 30 minutes. The clafoutis is ready when the custard has risen and is a golden color.

Remove from the oven, sprinkle with remaining herbs and serve immediately.

3 tbsp olive oil

2 onions, halved and thinly sliced

2 cloves garlic, coarsely chopped

1 rib celery, finely cubed

2 carrots, finely cubed

2fl oz/¼ cup/60ml water or vegetable stock

2fl oz/¼ cup/60ml white wine

2 tomatoes, chopped (or ½ 15 oz/400g jar of tomatoes) pinch of oregano

1.3lb/600 g firm white fish cut into steaks or fillets

10-12 coarsely chopped green or black olives

3 thin slices untreated lemon

2 tbsp chopped parsley salt & freshly ground black pepper

Greek fish and vegetable bake

One of the most popular ways of preparing fish in Greece, this dish (known as plaki) is eaten hot in winter, or lukewarm or cold as a refreshing summer meal. Leaving it to sit for a few hours after cooking allows the flavors to infuse and deepen.

Serves 4.

Preheat oven to 350°F/180°C.

In a medium pot soften the onions in the olive oil for 5 minutes. Add garlic, celery, carrots, water, wine, salt and pepper.

Cover and simmer for 10 minutes until the carrots are al dente, then add tomatoes and oregano and cook another 5 minutes, covered.

Lay fish steaks or fillets in a lightly oiled ovenproof dish, pour the sauce over it, scatter with chopped olives, lay lemon slices on top and cover with foil. Slide into oven and cook for

30 minutes or until the fish flakes easily when prodded with a sharp kitchen knife.

Remove from oven, leave to cool for 5 minutes (if eating hot), sprinkle with parsley and serve. Alternatively, cool and serve at room temperature.

Variation

For a complete meal, I sometimes place a layer of cooked

Garlicky spinach under the fish and bake the whole lot together.

1.3lb/2⅔ cups/600 g cooked French green lentils

2fl oz/¼ cup/60ml olive oil plus 3 tbsp

3 large eggplants cut into

6-7 mm slices

2 onions, sliced

2 cloves garlic, chopped

1¾ lb/800g tomatoes, cubed

1oz/25g dried porcini or shiitake mushrooms, rehydrated, drained and finely chopped

3.5fl oz/½ cup/120ml red wine

3 bay leaves

1 tsp thyme

1 tbsp each of oregano and mint

1 tsp cinnamon

13.5fl oz/1⅔ cups/400ml unsweetened soy or almond milk

2 tbsp whole wheat or spelt flour

2 tbsp olive oil

1 tsp turmeric pinch of grated nutmeg salt & pepper

This dish is inspired by the famous Greek Moussaka me melitzanes, but the name is where the similarity ends. First, I have replaced fatty lamb with nutty French green lentils.

Secondly, I do not sauté the eggplant slices in oil, but brush them lightly with olive oil and grill them, thus using much less oil and lightening up the dish. Serves 4-6.

Warm 2 tablespoons of the oil in a large pot on medium heat and gently cook onions and garlic until translucent (about 4-5 minutes). Add herbs and cinnamon, tomatoes, mushrooms and red wine and cook uncovered for 20 minutes until reduced by about one third; puree with a hand-held blender. Add cooked lentils to the tomato sauce and cook for another 15 minutes.

Remove from heat.

While the lentil sauce is cooking, lightly brush both sides of the eggplant slices with olive oil and place on a baking tray covered with baking parchment. Set grill on medium heat and grill eggplant slices on both sides until golden. Set aside.

For the béchamel topping, put cold milk, olive oil, flour, turmeric and nutmeg in a pot and whisk until combined. Set over medium heat and stir. After 2-3 minutes the mixture will start thickening; keep stirring until it bubbles gently. Cook another 1-2 minutes, stirring all the while. Remove from heat.

Lightly oil an ovenproof dish and get ready to layer. Start with a thin layer of lentil-tomato sauce followed by a layer of eggplant and continue in this way until you end with lentils on top.

Finish by pouring the béchamel over the pie and smoothing it out evenly with a spatula. Place in a preheated oven and cook for 15 minutes; sprinkle with crumbled feta cheese and cook another 10 minutes until the cheese is golden. Serve.

Lentil moussaka

7oz/1 cup/200g hulled barley, soaked for 12 hours and drained

2 tbsp olive oil

1 onion, finely chopped

4 cloves garlic, finelychopped

1.1lb/500g mushrooms (e.g. button, chestnut, oyster, shiitake), sliced

1oz/25g dried mushrooms, rehydrated in warm water for 15 minutes

½ tsp thyme

1⅔ pints/3 ½ cups/800ml vegetable or chicken stock

2-3 tbsp dry white wine

2 tbsp chopped parsley squeeze of lemon juice salt & freshly ground black pepper

1 tbsp butter grated Parmesan or pecorino cheese

Mushroom orzotto

A specialty from northern Italy, this is prepared like a classic risotto, only using barley (orzo in Italian) instead of rice. This substitution affords many advantages, for barley is rich in anti-cancer nutrients, such as selenium and lignans, as well as soluble fiber. It also has a lower GI rating than most types of rice. Barley needs to be soaked overnight; this makes it easier to digest and faster to cook. When buying barley, always choose hulled over pot or pearled barley which undergo more processing and are less nutritious. Serves 4.

In a large skillet on medium heat, warm a tablespoon of olive oil and cook garlic, fresh and rehydrated mushrooms and thyme, stirring regularly, until soft (about 10 minutes).

In a heavy-bottomed pot, heat another tablespoon olive oil on medium heat and gently cook the chopped onion, stirring regularly until it is translucent. Add barley and cook for a minute.

Now begin adding stock, ladle by ladle, and keep stirring while the barley grains slowly absorb the liquid.

After about 20 minutes of ladling and stirring you should have used up all the stock. The barley grains will have roughly doubled in volume and the mixture will be creamy. Now add cooked mushrooms and a splash of white wine and cook, stirring, for another 2-3 minutes. If the mixture appears too firm or sticky, add a little more stock, wine or water.

Test the grains: they should be soft but slightly chewy. Season with salt, pepper and lemon juice. Stir in the butter, transfer to a serving dish and sprinkle with grated cheese.

Variations

• For added protein, add cubed, firm tofu or leftover chicken.

• For a splash of color, stir in some baby spinach leaves, arugula or other fast-wilting greens a minute or two before serving.

1 onion, quartered and sliced

4 ribs celery, sliced

2 eggplants, diced

15oz/400g tomatoes, chopped

5 tbsp olive oil

12 black olives, sliced

2 tbsp red wine vinegar

1 tbsp acacia honey

2 tbsp capers

2 tbsp chopped basil or parsley

2 tbsp lightly toasted pine nuts salt & freshly ground black pepper

Sicilian eggplant stew

One of Sicily's best-known dishes is caponata, a delicious sweet-and-sour stew of meltingly soft eggplants, crunchy celery and pine nuts brought together by fruity tomatoes and rounded off with fragrant basil. Serves 4 as a side dish or hors d'oeuvre.

In a large, heavy-bottomed skillet, heat 2 tablespoons olive oil and cook onion and celery for 5 minutes, stirring regularly until translucent. Add eggplant cubes and remaining olive oil and continue cooking until the eggplant starts to turn golden (about 10 minutes), turning the vegetables occasionally with a spatula to prevent them sticking to the pan.

Add tomatoes, olives, vinegar, capers and honey and cover, simmering on a low heat for another 15 minutes. Just before serving, season to taste with salt and pepper, then sprinkle with basil and pine nuts.

This can be enjoyed warm or cold, on its own or accompanied by eggs, fish, lean meat or plain steamed bulgur or brown rice.

2 tbsp olive oil

1 onion, chopped

½ tsp gingerbread spice (or a generous pinch each of ginger, cloves, cinnamon and nutmeg)

1 tsp turmeric

1¾lb/800g tomatoes, chopped

3.5oz/⅔ cup/100g dried apricots, chopped

3 tbsp tomato paste

2 tbsp apple cider vinegar

1 tbsp acacia honey (optional) salt & freshly ground black pepper

Homemade tomato ketchup

If you think making your own ketchup is a little over-thetop, consider the advantages. Not only are you avoiding the drawbacks of mass-produced ketchup – excess sugar, salt and various additives. In addition, this ketchup enables you to consume small but regular doses of anti-cancer spices and foods throughout the day! Enjoy a small blob with your breakfast egg, another on your lunchbox sandwich and a third with fish or chicken for dinner – among countless other options. Makes about 2 pints/1l.

In a medium-sized pot on medium heat, gently cook the onion in olive oil until translucent. Add spices and cook for another minute, stirring continually.

Now add tomatoes, tomato paste, apricots, vinegar, salt and pepper. Bring to the boil, then reduce heat and cook for 30 minutes on the lowest setting. If using tomatoes from a jar, cover with a lid. If using fresh tomatoes (these generally contain more water), leave uncovered so that excess moisture can evaporate.

Transfer to a blender and liquidize to obtain a smooth, thick puree. If it is too thick, add a little water or apple juice. For an extra-smooth sauce, pass through a sieve. Season with a little more salt, vinegar and honey if necessary. Fill into an empty, thoroughly cleaned glass bottle. Wellsealed, this keeps in the refrigerator for at least two weeks.

2 eggs

4.5oz/1 ½ cups/125g ground almonds

4.5oz/1 cup/125g whole spelt or wheat flour

1 heaped tsp baking powder

1 tsp natural vanilla extract

10fl oz/1¼ cups/300ml milk (almond, hazelnut, soy or dairy) pinch of salt

Blueberry sauce

1.1lb/500g blueberries (fresh or defrosted) pinch of grated lemon zest (untreated)

3.5fl oz/scant ½ cup/100ml red berry juice

(e.g. blueberry, cherry, raspberry)

1 heaped tbsp corn starch mixed with 2-3 tbsp water or apple juice

2 tbsp honey

Almond waffles with blueberry sauce

For people trying to wean themselves off processed or starchy breakfast foods, here's a morning dish that's light yet filling and rich in healthy fats and protein to help stabilize bloodsugar levels. These can be made in advance, frozen (separated with small sheets of baking parchment) and defrosted under the grill. Makes 4-6 waffles, depending on the size of your waffle iron.

Start by making the blueberry sauce (this can be done in advance).

Combine juice and corn starch in a medium pot and bring to the boil; stir until the juice has thickened. Remove from heat, add blueberries, lemon zest and honey. Stir well and set aside to cool. Keeps for a week chilled in a tightly sealed container.

In a mixing bowl, combine all the waffle ingredients and whisk until you obtain a smooth, thick batter. Heat waffle iron and bake the waffles as directed by the machine's instructions. Cool for a minute on a wire rack and serve with the blueberry sauce.

Variations

• This recipe works equally well with ground hazelnuts in the place of almonds and 1 teaspoon cinnamon instead of vanilla extract. Topped with apple sauce, this makes a delicious winter breakfast.

• Add 1 tablespoon each of pure cocoa powder and honey to the batter for chocolate waffles.

1.1lb/500g mixed pitted cherries and berries (raspberries, strawberries, blueberries, cranberries, red- and blackcurrants, blackberries, gooseberries etc.), fresh or frozen

7fl oz/scant 1 cup/200ml cherry or red berry juice (or a combination of 4fl

oz/½ cup/120ml juice and

2.5fl oz/1/3 cup/80ml red wine for a more grownup version)

2 tbsp corn starch grated zest of ½ lemon (untreated)

3-4 tbsp acacia honey (more or less to taste) some mint leaves for decoration

Very berry summer pudding

It's hard to imagine a more concentrated – or delicious – way of enjoying our red, blue and purple friends, the berries and cherries. This is also a great way to get children to eat berries, which, on their own, they often find too tart. While it is best to eat fruits and vegetables during their local growing season, we can make an exception here: the berry season being woefully short and fresh berries often expensive, I'm happy to make this with frozen berries and enjoy it all year round. Serves 4.

If using frozen berries, scatter onto a large tray or platter and defrost (about 30 minutes).

Pour juice (or juice/wine mixture, whichever using) into a medium pot, add corn starch, lemon zest and honey and enjoy

mix. Over medium heat, bring the liquid to a simmer, stirring

continually with a balloon whisk until it thickens. Remove from

heat, tip in the defrosted berries and stir gently with a spoon to

coat these evenly with the thickened juice. Adjust sweetness with

honey, one spoonful at a time,

Spoon into a serving bowl (this looks particularly attractive in

a glass bowl) or individual glasses and cool. Decorate with mint

leaves and serve at room temperature or chilled.

If you like, you can serve this with Vanilla cashew cream or

topped with plain yogurt thinned with a little milk and flavored

with honey and vanilla.

Made in United States
Orlando, FL
24 February 2025